THE

SILENT KILLER

Uncovering the mysteries of heart disease

Esther C .Excel

Table of contents

INTRODUCTION

The Silent Killer: Uncovering the Mysteries of Heart Disease

Imagine a villain so cunning, it can strike without warning, leaving devastation in its wake. A villain so stealthy, it can masquerade as a harmless friend, only to reveal its true nature when it's too late. This is the story of heart disease, the silent killer that claims millions of lives worldwide each year.

Meet Sarah, a vibrant 45-year-old mother of two, who seemed to have it all together. She was a devoted wife, a loving parent, and a successful entrepreneur. But beneath the surface, a silent killer was lurking, waiting to strike. One fateful morning, Sarah woke up with a crushing chest pain, and her life was forever changed by a heart attack.

Or consider John, a 50-year-old marathon runner, who had always prided himself on his physical prowess. He was the epitome of health, or so he thought. But during a routine check-up, his doctor discovered a ticking time bomb - a severely blocked artery, threatening to unleash a deadly heart attack at any moment.

These stories illustrate the insidious nature of heart disease, a condition that can affect anyone, regardless of age, gender, or fitness level. It's a disease that can masquerade as fatigue, indigestion, or even a simple cold, only to reveal its true face when it's too late.

In this book, "The Silent Killer: Uncovering the Mysteries of Heart Disease," we'll embark on a journey to expose the truth behind this stealthy assassin. We'll delve into the mysteries of heart disease, exploring its causes, symptoms, and treatment options. We'll meet the heroes - doctors, researchers, and patients - fighting against this silent killer.

Through their stories, we'll uncover the intricate web of factors contributing to heart disease, from genetics and lifestyle choices to environmental factors and medical breakthroughs. We'll examine the latest research and innovations, offering hope and guidance for those affected by this condition.

This book is not just about heart disease; it's about the human spirit's capacity to overcome adversity. It's about the resilience of those who have faced the silent killer and emerged victorious. And it's about the power of knowledge, which can transform fear into empowerment.

So join me on this journey into the heart of darkness, where we'll confront the silent killer and emerge with a newfound understanding of this complex and mysterious disease. Together, let's uncover the truth and take control of our heart health.

CHAPTER 1: MYTHS AND MISCONCEPTIONS

Myths and Misconceptions: Separating Facts from Fiction

As we navigate the complex world of heart disease, it's easy to get caught up in a web of myths and misconceptions. These misconceptions can lead to confusion, misinformation, and even harm. In this chapter, we'll embark on a journey to separate fact from fiction, exploring the most common myths and misconceptions surrounding heart disease.

Meet Emily, a 30-year-old fitness enthusiast who thought she knew it all about heart health. She believed that heart disease only affected older, overweight people who didn't exercise. But when her mother, a healthy and active 55-year-old, suffered a heart attack, Emily's world was turned upside down.

"I was shocked," Emily said. "I thought my mom was the picture of health. I didn't realize that heart disease could affect anyone, regardless of age or fitness level."

Emily's story highlights one of the most common myths about heart disease: that it only affects older, unhealthy people. But the truth is, heart disease can affect anyone, at any age.

Myth 1: Heart Disease Only Affects Older People

Reality: Heart disease can affect anyone, regardless of age. While it's true that the risk increases with age, younger people can also be affected.

Myth 2: Heart Disease is a Man's Disease

Reality: Heart disease affects both men and women equally. Heart disease is the leading cause of death in women.

Myth 3: I'm Too Young for a Heart Attack

Reality: Heart attacks can occur at any age, even in young people. Family history, lifestyle choices, and underlying medical conditions can increase the risk.

Myth 4: I'm Fit, So I'm Safe

Reality: Fitness is important, but it's not a guarantee against heart disease. Other factors like genetics, diet, and stress levels also play a role.

Myth 5: Heart Disease is Inevitable

Reality: While some risk factors can't be changed, many can. Lifestyle choices like diet, exercise, and stress management can significantly reduce the risk of heart disease.

By separating fact from fiction, we can empower ourselves with knowledge and take control of our heart health. Remember, heart disease is a complex condition, and understanding the facts is crucial for prevention and treatment.

CHAPTER 2: THE HEART OF THE MATTER

Anatomy of the Heart: Understanding the Cardiovascular System

Meet Maya, a curious and ambitious medical student, eager to unravel the mysteries of the human body. As she delved into her studies, she became fascinated with the heart, a complex and vital organ that pumps life-giving blood throughout our bodies. Maya's journey took her deep into the anatomy of the heart, where she discovered a fascinating world of chambers, valves, and vessels.

We will be joining Maya on her journey, exploring the intricate details of the cardiovascular system. We'll venture into the heart's chambers, learn about the vital role of valves, and discover the extensive network of blood vessels that keep our bodies alive.

The Heart: A Muscular Marvel

The heart is a muscular organ, about the size of a fist, located in the thoracic cavity between the lungs. It's a remarkable structure, composed of four layers:

1. Epicardium: The outermost layer, a thin membrane that protects the heart.
2. Myocardium: The thick middle layer, made up of cardiac muscle cells that contract to pump blood.
3. Endocardium: The innermost layer, a thin membrane that lines the heart's chambers and valves.
4. Pericardium: A fibrous sac that surrounds and protects the heart.

Maya was amazed by the heart's muscular structure, capable of pumping over 2,000 gallons of blood daily. She learned that the heart beats around 100,000 times per day, a staggering 3 billion times in a lifetime.

Chambers of the Heart

The heart consists of four chambers:

1. Right Atrium (RA): Receives oxygen-depleted blood from the body.
2. Right Ventricle (RV): Pumps blood from the RA to the lungs.
3. Left Atrium (LA): Receives oxygen-rich blood from the lungs.

4. Left Ventricle (LV): Pumps blood from the LA to the rest of the body.

Maya visualized the chambers as a complex system, working together to circulate blood throughout the body.

Valves: The Heart's Guardians

Valves play a crucial role in regulating blood flow between the chambers. There are four valves:

1. Tricuspid Valve: Between the RA and RV.
2. Pulmonary Valve: Between the RV and lungs.
3. Mitral Valve: Between the LA and LV.
4. Aortic Valve: Between the LV and aorta.

Maya understood that valves ensure blood flows in one direction, preventing backflow and ensuring efficient circulation.

Blood Vessels: The Extensive Network

The cardiovascular system comprises:

1. Arteries: Carry oxygen-rich blood away from the heart.
2. Veins: Carry oxygen-depleted blood back to the heart.

3. Capillaries: Tiny vessels where oxygen and nutrients are exchanged.

Maya marveled at the vast network of blood vessels, spanning over 60,000 miles, more than twice the Earth's circumference.

Maya's journey through the anatomy of the heart and cardiovascular system left her in awe of the human body's complexity and beauty. She realized that understanding the heart's intricate details is crucial for appreciating its vital role in sustaining life.

Remember that the heart is a remarkable organ, deserving of our appreciation and care. By grasping its anatomy and functions, we can better comprehend the importance of heart health and take steps to protect this precious gift.

The Role of Genetics: Inheritance and Heart Disease

Meet Emma, a vibrant 28-year-old, who always thought she was invincible. Her life took a dramatic turn when her father, a seemingly healthy 55-year-old, suffered a sudden heart attack. Emma was shocked to learn that her father's heart disease was not just a result of his lifestyle choices, but also due to a genetic predisposition.

As Emma delved deeper into her family's medical history, she discovered a complex web of inherited traits that increased her own risk of heart disease.

The Genetic Blueprint

Genetics plays a significant role in shaping our risk of heart disease. Our DNA, the genetic blueprint, contains instructions for the development and function of our cardiovascular system. Emma learned that small variations in her DNA, known as genetic mutations, could affect her risk of heart disease.

Family History: A Powerful Predictor

Emma's family history revealed a pattern of heart disease, with multiple relatives affected at a young age. She realized that her father's heart attack was not just a coincidence, but a warning sign of her own increased risk.

The Role of Inherited Traits

The silent killer

Certain inherited traits can increase the risk of heart disease, including:

1. High blood pressure
2. High cholesterol
3. Diabetes
4. Obesity

Emma discovered that her family members had a history of these conditions, which significantly increased her own risk.

Genetic Mutations: The Culprits

Genetic mutations can affect the functioning of genes involved in heart health. Emma learned about the following mutations:

1. Familial Hypercholesterolemia (FH): A mutation that leads to extremely high cholesterol levels.
2. Hypertrophic Cardiomyopathy (HCM): A mutation that causes thickening of the heart muscle.

These mutations can increase the risk of heart disease, even in young people.

Epigenetics: The Environmental Influence

Epigenetics is the study of how environmental factors affect gene expression. Emma discovered that lifestyle choices, such as diet and exercise, can influence her genetic risk of heart disease.

The Interplay Between Genetics and Lifestyle

Emma learned that genetics and lifestyle are intertwined. While she couldn't change her genetic predisposition, she could modify her lifestyle to reduce her risk of heart disease.

Emma's journey through the world of genetics and heart disease revealed a complex interplay between inherited traits, genetic mutations, and lifestyle choices. She realized that understanding her genetic risk was crucial for taking proactive steps to protect her heart health.

Remember that genetics plays a significant role in heart disease, but it's not the sole determinant. By embracing a healthy lifestyle and understanding our genetic risk, we can empower ourselves to take control of our heart health.

Environmental Factors: Lifestyle Choices and Heart Health

Meet Jack, a 45-year-old successful businessman, who always prioritized his career over his health. He spent long hours at work, fueled by coffee and fast food, and rarely exercised. Jack's lifestyle choices eventually caught up with him, and he suffered a heart attack at the age of 50.

As Jack recovered, he realized that his lifestyle choices had significantly contributed to his heart disease. He began to explore the impact of environmental factors on heart health and made significant changes to his daily habits.

We'll join Jack on his journey, examining the intricate relationship between environmental factors, lifestyle choices, and heart health.

The Impact of Diet

Jack's diet was a major contributor to his heart disease. He consumed high amounts of:

1. Saturated fats
2. Sodium

3. Refined sugars

These dietary choices increased his risk of heart disease by:

1. Raising cholesterol levels
2. Increasing blood pressure
3. Promoting inflammation

Jack learned that a heart-healthy diet rich in:

1. Fruits
2. Vegetables
3. Whole grains
4. Lean proteins

Could help mitigate these risks.

The Importance of Exercise

Jack's sedentary lifestyle also played a significant role in his heart disease. Regular exercise can:

1. Lower blood pressure
2. Improve lipid profiles
3. Reduce inflammation

Jack started with small changes, such as:

1. Taking the stairs instead of the elevator
2. Walking during his lunch break
3. Gradually increasing his physical activity

Stress Management

Chronic stress can significantly impact heart health by:

1. Increasing blood pressure
2. Promoting inflammation
3. Disrupting sleep patterns

Jack learned stress management techniques, such as:

1. Meditation
2. Yoga
3. Deep breathing exercises

Sleep and Heart Health

Poor sleep quality and duration can increase the risk of heart disease by:

1. Disrupting stress hormones
2. Increasing inflammation
3. Affecting lipid profiles

Jack prioritized sleep, aiming for 7-8 hours per night, and established a relaxing bedtime routine.

Jack's journey highlights the significant impact of environmental factors and lifestyle choices on heart health. By making informed choices, we can reduce our risk of heart disease and promote overall well-being.

Remember, small changes can add up over time. Start with:

1. Healthy eating habits
2. Regular exercise
3. Stress management techniques
4. Prioritizing sleep

Take control of your heart health today!

CHAPTER 3: THE MYSTERIES OF HEART DISEASE

The Enigma of Atherosclerosis: Uncovering the Causes

Dr. Maria, a renowned cardiologist, had always been fascinated by the complexities of atherosclerosis. She had spent years studying the condition, but still, the exact causes remained an enigma. One patient, in particular, caught her attention - a young and seemingly healthy 35-year-old, who had suffered a sudden heart attack.

As Dr. Maria delved deeper into the patient's case, she began to unravel the mysteries of atherosclerosis. She discovered that the condition was not just a result of high cholesterol or smoking, but a complex interplay of factors.

Let's join Dr. Maria on her journey, exploring the intricate causes of atherosclerosis.

The Role of Inflammation

Dr. Maria learned that inflammation played a crucial role in the development of atherosclerosis. The patient's blood tests revealed high levels of inflammatory markers, which indicated an immune response gone awry.

The Impact of Oxidative Stress

Oxidative stress, a state of imbalance between free radicals and antioxidants, was another key player in the patient's condition. Dr. Maria discovered that the patient's diet was lacking essential antioxidants, making him more susceptible to oxidative stress.

The Influence of Genetics

Dr. Maria explored the patient's family history and discovered a pattern of early-onset heart disease. This led her to suspect a genetic component, which was later confirmed through genetic testing.

The Role of Lipids

Dr. Maria examined the patient's lipid profile and found high levels of low-density lipoprotein (LDL) cholesterol and triglycerides. She explained to the patient that these lipids could accumulate in the arterial walls, leading to plaque formation.

The Impact of Lifestyle Choices

Dr. Maria discussed the patient's lifestyle choices, including a diet high in processed foods, lack of exercise, and stress. She emphasized that these choices had contributed to his increased risk of atherosclerosis.

The Interplay of Factors

Dr. Maria realized that atherosclerosis was not caused by a single factor, but rather an interplay of genetic, environmental, and lifestyle factors. She explained to the patient that addressing these factors could help prevent further progression of the disease.

Dr. Maria's journey with her patient highlighted the complexities of atherosclerosis. By uncovering the causes, she was able to develop a comprehensive treatment plan, that addressed the patient's unique needs.

Remember, atherosclerosis is a multifactorial condition, requiring a holistic approach. By understanding the interplay of factors, we can take proactive steps to prevent and manage this condition.

The Inflammation Connection: How the Body's Response Contributes

Sarah, a vibrant and active 40-year-old, suddenly found herself struggling with chronic fatigue, joint pain, and brain fog. She had always been healthy, but now her body seemed to be turning against her. After months of testing, Sarah was diagnosed with rheumatoid arthritis, an autoimmune disease characterized by chronic inflammation.

As Sarah delved deeper into her condition, she discovered a fascinating yet complex world of inflammation. She learned that inflammation was not just a symptom, but a vital response of the body's immune system. In this chapter, we'll join Sarah on her journey, exploring the intricate connection between inflammation and disease.

The Inflammation Response

Inflammation is the body's natural defense against injury or infection. When the immune system detects harm, it triggers an inflammatory response, sending white blood cells to fight off the invader. This response is essential for healing and protection.

However, when inflammation becomes chronic, it can lead to devastating consequences. Sarah's rheumatoid arthritis was a prime example, where her immune system mistakenly attacked her joints, causing inflammation and damage.

The Role of Cytokines

Cytokines are signaling molecules that facilitate communication between immune cells. They play a crucial role in initiating and maintaining inflammation. Sarah discovered that cytokines like TNF-alpha and IL-6 were key players in her rheumatoid arthritis, promoting inflammation and joint damage.

The Impact of Oxidative Stress

Oxidative stress occurs when the body's antioxidant defenses are overwhelmed by free radicals. This imbalance can trigger inflammation and damage tissues. Sarah learned that oxidative stress was a key contributor to her rheumatoid arthritis, as well as an independent risk factor for other diseases.

The Gut Connection

The gut microbiome plays a vital role in regulating inflammation and immune responses. Sarah discovered that an imbalance of gut bacteria, known as dysbiosis, was contributing to her chronic inflammation and rheumatoid arthritis.

The Mind-Body Connection

Sarah learned that stress and emotions can also contribute to inflammation. Chronic stress can lead to increased levels of cortisol, a hormone that promotes inflammation. Additionally, negative emotions like anxiety and depression can exacerbate inflammation.

The Role of Nutrition

Sarah discovered that her diet was a significant contributor to her inflammation. She learned that a diet high in processed foods, sugar, and unhealthy fats can promote inflammation, while a diet rich in fruits, vegetables, and omega-3 fatty acids can help reduce it.

Sarah's journey through the world of inflammation revealed a complex web of relationships between her immune system, inflammation, and disease. She learned that chronic inflammation was not just a symptom, but a driving force behind her rheumatoid arthritis and other diseases.

By understanding the intricate connections between inflammation, immune responses, and disease, we can take proactive steps to mitigate risk and promote overall well-being. Remember, inflammation is a double-edged sword - essential for healing, but devastating when chronic. Take control of your inflammation today!

The Role of Hormones: Balancing the Body's Chemicals

Meet Emily, a 30-year-old fitness enthusiast, who has always been passionate about living a healthy lifestyle. However, despite her best efforts, she began to experience unexplained weight gain, fatigue, and mood swings. After months of frustration, Emily discovered that her hormone levels were out of balance.

We'll join Emily on her journey, exploring the intricate world of hormones and their role in maintaining the body's delicate balance.

The Hormone System

Hormones are chemical messengers produced by glands in the endocrine system. They regulate various bodily functions, including growth, metabolism, and reproductive processes. Emily learned that even small imbalances in hormone levels could have significant effects on her overall health.

The Role of Insulin

Insulin, produced by the pancreas, regulates blood sugar levels. Emily discovered that her insulin resistance was contributing to her weight gain and fatigue. She learned that a balanced diet and regular exercise could help improve insulin sensitivity.

The Impact of Thyroid Hormones

Thyroid hormones, produced by the thyroid gland, regulate metabolism. Emily's hypothyroidism was causing her fatigue, weight gain, and mood swings. She learned that thyroid hormone replacement therapy could help restore balance.

The Influence of Adrenal Hormones

Adrenal hormones, produced by the adrenal glands, regulate stress response. Emily's chronic stress was leading to adrenal fatigue, causing her to feel exhausted and burnt out. She learned that stress management techniques, such as meditation and yoga, could help reduce cortisol levels.

The Role of Sex Hormones

Sex hormones, including estrogen and testosterone, regulate reproductive processes. Emily's hormonal birth control was disrupting her natural balance, leading to mood swings and weight gain. She learned that alternative methods, such as natural family planning, could help restore balance.

The Interplay of Hormones

Emily discovered that hormones work together in a delicate balance. For example, insulin resistance can lead to increased androgen levels, causing acne and hair loss. She learned that addressing one hormonal imbalance could have a ripple effect, improving overall hormone balance.

Emily's journey through the world of hormones revealed a complex web of relationships between her body's chemicals. She learned that hormonal balance is essential for maintaining overall health and well-being.

By understanding the intricate role of hormones, we can take proactive steps to promote balance and mitigate the risk of hormonal imbalances. Remember, hormones are the body's chemical messengers - essential for maintaining harmony within. Take control of your hormones today!

CHAPTER 4: DETECTION AND DIAGNOSIS.

Recognizing the Signs: Symptoms and Warning Signs

Meet Rachel, a busy working mom, who had always prioritized her family's health over her own. However, when she started experiencing persistent fatigue, shortness of breath, and chest pain, she knew something was wrong. After months of dismissing her symptoms, Rachel finally visited her doctor, only to discover that she was on the verge of a heart attack.

We'll join Rachel on her journey, exploring the often subtle signs and symptoms of heart disease. We'll delve into the warning signs that Rachel ignored and the importance of recognizing them early.

The Silent Killer

Heart disease is often referred to as a silent killer because its symptoms can be subtle and easy to ignore. Rachel's fatigue, for example, was dismissed as exhaustion from work and family responsibilities. However, fatigue is a common symptom of heart disease, especially in women.

The Warning Signs

Rachel's shortness of breath was another warning sign she ignored. She attributed it to being out of shape, but shortness of breath can be a sign of heart failure or coronary artery disease.

Chest pain is a classic symptom of heart disease, but Rachel's chest pain was intermittent and not severe enough to raise alarm bells. However, chest pain can manifest differently in women, often feeling like a squeezing sensation or tightness.

Other warning signs that Rachel ignored included:

- Swelling in her legs and feet
- Lightheadedness and dizziness
- Palpitations and irregular heartbeat

The Importance of Recognizing Signs Early

Rachel's story highlights the importance of recognizing the signs and symptoms of heart disease early. By ignoring her warning signs, Rachel put herself at risk of a heart attack.

If you're experiencing any of the following symptoms, don't ignore them:

- Chest pain or discomfort
- Shortness of breath
- Fatigue or weakness
- Swelling in your legs, ankles, or feet
- Lightheadedness or dizziness
- Palpitations or irregular heartbeat

Rachel's journey serves as a reminder that heart disease can affect anyone, regardless of age or health status. By recognizing the signs and symptoms early, we can take proactive steps to prevent heart disease and reduce the risk of heart attacks.

Remember, heart disease is a treatable condition, but only if we acknowledge the warning signs and take action. Don't ignore your body's signals - listen to them and take control of your heart health today!

Diagnostic Tools: Tests and Procedures for Heart Disease.

Michael,v is a 55-year-old entrepreneur, who has always been driven to succeed. However, when he started experiencing chest pain and shortness of breath, he knew something was wrong. Michael's doctor ordered a series of tests to determine the cause of his symptoms. In this chapter, we'll follow Michael's journey, exploring the diagnostic tools used to detect heart disease.

Electrocardiogram (ECG or EKG)

Michael's first test was an electrocardiogram, which measures the heart's electrical activity. The ECG revealed that Michael's heart was beating irregularly, indicating a possible heart rhythm disorder.

Echocardiogram

Next, Michael underwent an echocardiogram, which uses sound waves to create images of the heart. The test showed that Michael's heart was pumping inefficiently, suggesting heart failure.

Stress Test

Michael's doctor ordered a stress test to assess his heart's function under physical stress. The test revealed that Michael's heart was not receiving enough blood flow during exercise, indicating coronary artery disease.

Blood Tests

Michael's blood tests showed high levels of troponin, a protein released when the heart is damaged. This confirmed that Michael had suffered a heart attack.

Cardiac Catheterization

Michael underwent cardiac catheterization, a procedure that uses a catheter to inject dye into the coronary arteries. The test revealed blockages in Michael's arteries, confirming coronary artery disease.

Cardiac MRI

Finally, Michael had a cardiac MRI, which provided detailed images of his heart. The test showed scarring on Michael's heart, indicating previous heart damage.

Michael's journey highlights the importance of diagnostic tools in detecting heart disease. By undergoing these tests and procedures, Michael's doctor was able to diagnose his condition and develop an effective treatment plan.

Remember, if you're experiencing symptoms or have concerns about your heart health, consult a doctor or healthcare professional for personalized advice. They will determine the appropriate diagnostic tools and tests to assess your heart health.

The Importance of Early Detection: Why Timing Matters

Emma, a vibrant 40-year-old, who had always prioritized her health. However, when she started experiencing mild chest discomfort, she dismissed it as stress. Weeks later, Emma's symptoms worsened, and she visited her doctor. Timely detection revealed a heart condition, and Emma's life was forever changed.

The Power of Prevention

Emma's story emphasizes the significance of prevention. Regular check-ups and screenings can identify risk factors before symptoms appear. By addressing these risks early, individuals can prevent heart disease from developing or progressing.

The Window of Opportunity

Early detection offers a window of opportunity for effective treatment. When Emma's condition was diagnosed, her doctor was able to prescribe medication and lifestyle changes to manage her symptoms. If left undetected, Emma's condition could have progressed, reducing treatment options.

The Impact of Delayed Detection

Delayed detection can have devastating consequences. Heart disease can progress silently, and symptoms may only appear when the condition is advanced. In such cases, treatment options may be limited, and outcomes less favorable.

The Role of Awareness

Awareness plays a crucial role in early detection. Emma's knowledge of heart health and her body's signals enabled her to seek medical attention. Educating oneself about heart disease, its risk factors, and its symptoms can empower individuals to take control of their heart health.

The Importance of Screening

Screening tests, such as blood pressure checks, cholesterol screenings, and electrocardiograms, can detect heart disease early. Emma's doctor had recommended regular screenings, which ultimately led to her timely diagnosis.

Emma's journey highlights the importance of early detection in heart health. By prioritizing prevention, being aware of one's body, and undergoing regular screenings, individuals can ensure timely detection and effective treatment.

Remember, if you're experiencing symptoms or have concerns about your heart health, consult a doctor or healthcare professional for personalized advice. They will determine the appropriate course of action to address your specific needs.

CHAPTER 5: TREATMENT AND MANAGEMENT

Conventional Treatment: Medications and Surgical Options

Meet David, a 50-year-old businessman, who had been living with heart disease for years. Despite his best efforts to manage his condition through lifestyle changes, David's symptoms worsened, and his doctor recommended conventional treatment. Let's follow David's journey as he explores medications and surgical options.

Medications

David's doctor prescribed a combination of medications to manage his symptoms and slow disease progression. These included:

- Beta-blockers to reduce blood pressure and heart rate

- Statins to lower cholesterol levels
- ACE inhibitors to relax blood vessels
- Antiplatelet agents to prevent blood clots

David learned about potential side effects and interactions, and his doctor monitored him closely.

Surgical Options

As David's condition advanced, his doctor recommended surgical options. David underwent:

- Coronary artery bypass grafting (CABG) to restore blood flow
- Angioplasty and stenting to open blocked arteries
- Heart valve repair or replacement to address valve damage

David understood the risks and benefits of each procedure and worked closely with his doctor to determine the best course of action.

Device Therapy

David's doctor also recommended device therapy, including:

- Pacemakers to regulate heart rhythm

- Implantable cardioverter-defibrillators (ICDs) to prevent sudden cardiac death
- Cardiac resynchronization therapy (CRT) to improve heart function

David learned about device management and maintenance.

Lifestyle Changes

Throughout his treatment, David continued to prioritize lifestyle changes, including:

- Healthy eating habits
- Regular exercise
- Stress management
- Getting enough sleep

David's journey highlights the importance of conventional treatment in managing heart disease. By combining medications, surgical options, device therapy, and lifestyle changes, David effectively managed his symptoms and slowed disease progression.

Remember, if you're living with heart disease, consult a doctor or healthcare professional to determine the best treatment plan for your specific needs.

Alternative Approaches: Lifestyle Changes and Supplements

Meet Sarah, a 40-year-old yoga instructor, who had always prioritized natural health. When her mother was diagnosed with heart disease, Sarah sought alternative approaches to support her mother's recovery. In this chapter, we'll follow Sarah's journey as she explores lifestyle changes and supplements.

Lifestyle Changes

Sarah's mother began by adopting lifestyle changes, including:

- A plant-based diet rich in fruits, vegetables, and whole grains
- Regular yoga practice to reduce stress and improve circulation
- Quitting smoking and limiting alcohol consumption
- Getting enough sleep and practicing relaxation techniques

Supplements

Sarah's mother also incorporated supplements into her daily routine, including:

- Omega-3 fatty acids to reduce inflammation
- Coenzyme Q10 (CoQ10) to improve energy production
- Vitamin D to support heart health
- Turmeric/Curcumin to reduce inflammation

Sarah learned about potential interactions and consulted with a healthcare professional to ensure safe usage.

Stress Management

Sarah's mother practiced stress-reducing techniques, including:

- Meditation
- Deep breathing exercises
- Yoga Nidra
- Journaling

These practices helped manage stress and promote overall well-being.

Social Support

Sarah's mother surrounded herself with a supportive community, including:

- Family and friends

- Support groups
- Online forums

Social connections played a vital role in her recovery.

Mind-Body Connection

Sarah's mother explored the mind-body connection, recognizing that emotional well-being impacts physical health. She practiced:

- Gratitude journaling
- Positive affirmations
- Creative expression

This holistic approach supported her overall health.

Sarah's journey highlights the importance of alternative approaches in supporting heart health. By combining lifestyle changes, supplements, stress management, social support, and mind-body connection, Sarah's mother effectively managed her heart disease.

Remember, if you're considering alternative approaches, consult a healthcare professional to determine the best course of action for your specific needs.

Managing Heart Disease: Creating a Personalized Plan

Mark, a 55-year-old entrepreneur, had been living with heart disease for years. After a recent heart attack, Mark's doctor emphasized the importance of creating a personalized plan to manage his condition. We'll follow Mark's journey as he develops a tailored plan to take control of his heart health.

Setting Goals

Mark started by setting realistic goals, including:

- Reducing his blood pressure
- Lowering his cholesterol levels
- Increasing his physical activity
- Managing stress

Assessing Risk Factors

Mark worked with his doctor to identify his risk factors, including:

- Family history
- High blood pressure
- High cholesterol
- Smoking

Developing a Plan

Mark's doctor helped him create a personalized plan, including:

- Medications to manage blood pressure and cholesterol
- A customized exercise program
- Stress management techniques
- Dietary changes

Monitoring Progress

Mark regularly monitored his progress, tracking:

- Blood pressure
- Cholesterol levels
- Blood glucose levels
- Physical activity

Adjusting the Plan

As Mark's needs changed, his doctor adjusted his plan, including:

- Medication changes
- Exercise modifications
- Dietary adjustments

Lifestyle Changes

Mark made significant lifestyle changes, including:

- Quitting smoking
- Reducing alcohol consumption
- Getting enough sleep
- Practicing relaxation techniques

Support System

Mark surrounded himself with a supportive network, including:

- Family and friends
- Support groups
- Online forums

Mark's journey highlights the importance of creating a personalized plan to manage heart disease. By setting goals, assessing risk factors, developing a plan, monitoring progress, adjusting the plan, making lifestyle changes, and building a support system, Mark took control of his heart health.

CHAPTER 6: PREVENTION AND FUTURE DIRECTIONS

Preventing Heart Disease: Strategies for a Healthy Heart

Meet Sophia, a 35-year-old marketing executive, who had always been driven to succeed. However, when her mother suffered a heart attack, Sophia realized that she needed to prioritize her heart health. In this chapter, we'll follow Sophia's journey as she learns about preventing heart disease and adopts strategies for a healthy heart.

Understanding Risk Factors

Sophia's first step was to understand her risk factors. She learned that family history, age, gender, and ethnicity all play a role. She also discovered that lifestyle choices, such as diet, exercise, and stress levels, significantly impact heart health.

Healthy Eating Habits

Sophia started by revamping her diet. She focused on consuming:

- Leafy greens
- Berries
- Nuts
- Fatty fish
- Whole grains

She limited her intake of:

- Processed foods
- Sugary drinks
- Saturated fats

Regular Exercise

Sophia incorporated physical activity into her daily routine, aiming for:

- 150 minutes of moderate exercise
- 75 minutes of vigorous exercise
- Strength training exercises

Stress Management

Sophia learned stress management techniques, including:

- Meditation
- Yoga
- Deep breathing exercises

Getting Enough Sleep

Sophia prioritized sleep, aiming for 7-8 hours per night. She established a relaxing bedtime routine to improve sleep quality.

Monitoring and Maintaining

Sophia regularly monitored her:

- Blood pressure
- Cholesterol levels
- Blood glucose levels

She worked with her doctor to maintain healthy levels and address any concerns.

Sophia's journey highlights the importance of preventing heart disease through lifestyle changes. By understanding risk factors, adopting healthy habits, and regularly monitoring her health, Sophia significantly reduced her risk of heart disease.

Remember, if you're concerned about your heart health, consult a doctor or healthcare professional for personalized advice. They will help you develop a plan tailored to your specific needs.

Emerging Research: New Frontiers in Heart Disease Treatment

Dr. Patel, a renowned cardiologist, had dedicated her career to finding innovative solutions for heart disease. She was fascinated by the latest research in gene therapy, stem cell therapy, and nanotechnology. In this chapter, we'll explore the exciting new frontiers in heart disease treatment through Dr. Patel's journey.

Gene Therapy

Dr. Patel was particularly interested in gene therapy, which involves modifying genes to prevent or treat heart disease. She studied the use of viral vectors to deliver healthy copies of a gene to damaged heart cells, promoting regeneration.

Stem Cell Therapy

Dr. Patel also explored stem cell therapy, which harnesses the power of stem cells to repair damaged heart tissue. She investigated the use of induced pluripotent stem cells (iPSCs) to create personalized heart cells for transplantation.

Nanotechnology

Dr. Patel was intrigued by nanotechnology's potential to revolutionize heart disease treatment. She researched nanoparticles that could target specific cells, delivering medications or genetic material to precise locations.

Tissue Engineering

Dr. Patel investigated tissue engineering, which involves creating artificial heart tissue to replace damaged areas. She studied biomaterials and 3D printing techniques to create functional heart tissue.

Precision Medicine

Dr. Patel was excited about precision medicine, which tailors treatment to an individual's unique genetic profile. She explored genetic testing and personalized therapies to optimize heart disease treatment.

Dr. Patel's journey highlights the promising new frontiers in heart disease treatment. Emerging research in gene therapy, stem cell therapy, nanotechnology, tissue engineering, and precision medicine offers hope for more effective and personalized treatments.

Remember, while these advancements show promise, consult a doctor or healthcare professional for accurate information and guidance as health differs in individuals.

CONCLUSION

Taking Control of Your Heart Health

Meet Rachel, a 45-year-old mother of two, who has been living with heart disease for years. After experiencing a wake-up call, Rachel decided to take control of her heart health. In this final chapter, we'll follow Rachel's journey as she reflects on her experiences and shares her insights on taking control of your heart health.

Reflecting on the Journey

Rachel looked back on her journey, remembering the fear and uncertainty that came with her diagnosis. She recalled the struggles of managing her condition, the setbacks, and the triumphs. Through it all, Rachel learned valuable lessons about resilience, self-care, and the importance of taking control.

Empowerment Through Knowledge

Rachel emphasized the importance of education in managing heart disease. She encouraged others to learn about their condition, treatment options, and lifestyle changes. By being informed, individuals can make empowered decisions about their care.

Self-Care and Support

Rachel stressed the significance of self-care and support in heart health management. She encouraged others to prioritize activities that bring joy, practice stress-reducing techniques, and build a strong support network.

Mindset Shift

Rachel shared her own mindset shift, from feeling helpless to taking control. She encouraged others to adopt a growth mindset, focusing on progress, not perfection.

Rachel's journey serves as a testament to the power of taking control of your heart health. By educating yourself, prioritizing self-care, and adopting a growth mindset, you can manage your condition and improve your overall well-being.

Remember, heart disease is a manageable condition. Take control of your heart health today.

Note: Please consult a medical professional for personalized advice and diagnosis.

This concludes our journey through the world of heart health. We hope you found this story informative, engaging, and empowering. Remember, taking control of your heart health is a journey, and every step counts.

APPENDIX

Glossary of terms

1. **Atherosclerosis**: The buildup of plaque in the arteries, leading to hardening and narrowing.

2. **Angina**: Chest pain or discomfort due to reduced blood flow to the heart.

3. **Arrhythmia**: Abnormal heart rhythm.

4. **Blood Pressure**: The force of blood against artery walls.

5. **Cardiac Arrest**: Sudden loss of heart function.

6. **Cardiomyopathy**: Disease of the heart muscle.

7. **Cholesterol**: A fatty substance in the blood.

8. **Coronary Artery Disease (CAD):** Narrowing of the coronary arteries.

9. **Electrocardiogram** (ECG or EKG): Measures the heart's electrical activity.

10. **Heart Failure**: Inability of the heart to pump enough blood.

11. **Hypertension**: High blood pressure.

12. **Lipids**: Fats and cholesterol in the blood.

13. **Myocardial Infarction** (MI): Heart attack.

14. **Palpitations**: Irregular heartbeats.

15. **Peripheral Artery Disease (PAD):** Narrowing of peripheral arteries.

16. **Statins**: Medications to lower cholesterol.

17. **Stent**: A device to keep arteries open.

18. **Stroke**: Loss of brain function due to lack of blood supply.

19. **Tachycardia**: Rapid heart rate.

20. **Triglycerides**: A type of fat in the blood.

Resources for further learning

Here are some resources for further learning about heart disease:

Websites:

1. American Heart Association (AHA)
2. American College of Cardiology (ACC)
3. Centers for Disease Control and Prevention (CDC)
4. National Heart, Lung, and Blood Institute (NHLBI)
5. Mayo Clinic

Books:

1. "The Heart Disease Prevention and Reversal Program" by Dr. Dean Ornish
2. "Prevent and Reverse Heart Disease" by Dr. Caldwell Esselstyn
3. "The Cardiac Recovery Handbook" by Dr. David S. Feldman
4. "Heart 411" by Dr. Marc Gillinov and Dr. Steven Nissen
5. "The Heart Health Bible" by Dr. John M. Kennedy

Journals:

1. Journal of the American College of Cardiology (JACC)
2. Circulation
3. Heart
4. European Heart Journal
5. American Journal of Cardiology

Online Courses:

1. Coursera - "Heart Disease" by University of California, Irvine
2. edX - "Cardiovascular Disease" by Harvard University
3. Udemy - "Heart Disease Prevention and Management"

Support Groups:

1. American Heart Association Support Network
2. Heart Failure Support Network
3. WomenHeart: The National Coalition for Women with Heart Disease

References

Here are some other references that may be useful for heart disease:

1. American Heart Association. (2022). Heart Disease and Stroke Statistics—2022 Update.

2. Centers for Disease Control and Prevention. (2022). Heart Disease.

3. Mayo Clinic. (2022). Heart disease.

4. National Institute of Health. (2022). Heart Disease.

5. World Health Organization. (2022). Cardiovascular diseases.

6. European Society of Cardiology. (2022). Guidelines for the management of acute coronary syndromes.

7. American College of Cardiology. (2022). Guidelines for the management of heart failure.

8. Journal of the American College of Cardiology.

9. Circulation: Journal of the American Heart Association.

10. European Heart Journal.

Remember to consult a medical professional for personalized advice and diagnosis.